THE KETO DIET BOOK FOR BEGINNERS

Lose Weight with Quick and Delicious Recipes For Everyone incl. Vegan and Vegetarian Recipes

Sarah C. Smith

ISBN - 9798654218650

TABLE OF CONTENTS

3

INTRODUCTION

WHAT IS KETO DIET?

The classic ketogenic diet includes very low carbohydrate meals that have been used by researchers at Johns Hopkins Medical Center since the 1980s to treat epilepsy.

In a classic ketogenic diet, you limit the consumption of all foods containing sugar and carbohydrates. When we eat these foods, they break down into sugar in the blood, and if they are consumed more than usual intake of body, excess calories are stored in the body as fat, resulting in unwanted weight gain. However, once sugar levels drop with low sugar intake, the body begins to burn fat and turn out ketones.

The ketogenic diet works like most of the low carbohydrate diets by way of eliminating glucose. Most people often consume high carbohydrates, making glucose the primary source of energy that the body uses. We are unable to produce glucose, and we can only store it for up to 3 hours in the muscle and liver. When glucose is unavailable, our body will use stored fats or fats in foods instead.

Our body burns more fat as energy by following a ketogenic diet. The reason for the speedy weight loss and dehydration of fats following the ketogenic diet is the use of fat as a fuel supply. Even this weight loss occurs when you are not restricting calories and consuming high fat. Another vital advantage of a keto diet is that you just won't feel hungry and don't have to be compelled to count calories and do several hours of high-intensity exercise to burn calories.

In some respects, the ketogenic diet is just like the Atkins weight loss program. In these two diets, you can burn fat by limiting sugar and carbohydrates while using low carbohydrate foods. By eliminating the glucose obtained from foods, your body uses fat as an energy source. The ketogenic diet emphasizes the intake of healthy fats, less protein, and the elimination of processed meats, which also have strong scientific evidence.

With a ketogenic diet, you enter a phase called "ketosis," which occurs when the body is supplied with ketones instead of glucose. The ketosis phase is the opposite of the glucose state, where glucose provides the body with energy.

Here you can see benefits of Keto Diet

1. Automatic weight loss

Weight loss within the ketogenic diet is an inherent associated issue, particularly in corpulent and overweight individuals. A recent study by British people Journal of Nutrition found that individuals within the ketogenic diet had higher weight loss and a lower risk of cardiovascular disease compared to those in the diet.

Also, 6 years studying on keto diet confirmed that:

One of the diets that have been studied for weight loss in recent years is the ketogenic diet. Many studies show that this style has a strong biochemical and basic physiological nutrition that's capable of effective weight loss in conjunction with an improvement in many parameters of cardiovascular diseases.

The ketogenic diet affects weight loss and appetite because of its high fat, low carbohydrate and hormonal effects. As mentioned above, eating less of our carbohydrates will produce less insulin. Lower insulin levels mean you're not storing energy within the sort of fat associated. You are ready to consume fat reserves as an energy supply.

The ketogenic diet is highly nutritious due to its high content of healthy fats and high-quality protein that prevents over-eating nutritious, sugary and empty calories. For most people, having a low-carbohydrate diet makes it easy for them to get enough calories and also eliminates sugary drinks, cookies, bread and breakfast cereals, ice cream and desserts.

Polycystic ovary syndrome is one among the foremost common endocrine disorders that have an effect on the fertility of girls. Symptoms of obesity include hyperinsulinemia and insulin resistance. One study was conducted on 3 women for 5 weeks in which they were on a ketogenic diet with less than 1 g carbohydrate per day. At the end of the study, women experienced, on average 1% weight loss and 2% fasting insulin. Also, the two women had a history of infertility and could become pregnant.

2. Reduces Type 1 diabetes risk

The benefits of a ketogenic diet are far beyond fat burning. The ketogenic diet has helped to regulate the release of hormones such as insulin, which play a role in diabetes production and other health issues. With carbohydrate intake, blood glucose levels rise and insulin is released in response to it, Insulin is a storage hormone that sends signals to cells to store energy as much as possible, at first this energy is stored as glycogen in the muscles and then stored as body fat.

Studies have shown that the ketogenic diet is beneficial for improving blood pressure and insulin secretion.

3. Reduce the risk of heart disease

The ketogenic diet reduces the symptoms of heart disease, including triglycerides and high cholesterol. In fact, despite being high in fat, the ketogenic diet does not harm cholesterol levels. In addition, the keto diet is able to lower cardiovascular disease factors, especially in obese individuals.

4. Reduce the Risk of Cancer

One research showed that following a ketogenic diet and using foods within the ketogenic diet for three weeks reduced levels of triglycerides, LDL cholesterol, and blood sugar considerably in patients. HDL cholesterol levels were also elevated at the same time.

Studies have suggested that the ketogenic diet destroys cancer cells. Processed foods with very low nutritional value can nourish cancer cells.

What is the relationship between high sugar consumption and cancer?

Normal cells in our body are able to use fat as associate energy supply, however, researchers believe that cancer cells metabolically cannot use fat rather than glucose.

Several medical studies have shown that a ketogenic diet is an efficient treatment for cancer and other serious health issues.

The ketogenic diet is an effective way to reduce cancer by removing sugars and refined carbohydrates. **It's no coincidence that a number of the best cancer-fighting foods are on the ketogenic food list.**

5. Fight against brain diseases and neurological disorders

Over the last century, the keto diet has been used as a natural treatment and even to relieve neurological disorders and cognitive impairments such as Alzheimer's, epilepsy, anxiety and severe depression. Research shows that minimizing glucose levels using a ketogenic diet will force your body to produce ketones for fuel. This alteration of the body's fuel can eliminate cognitive impairments and neurological disorders, including epileptic seizures. The brain is in a position to use this alternative fuel instead of the usual method (using glucose as fuel), which does not work properly in patients with cerebral condition patients.

Published reports show that while diseases are different, the ketogenic diet is effective for Several neurological disorders because it has nerve-protective effects.

Also, an experiment on mice showed that the ketogenic diet slows down the process of ESL and Huntington's disease.

Scientists also claim that the ketogenic diet helps schizophrenic patients to recover from symptoms such as hallucinations and unpredictable behaviours. Although it is unclear the exact role of ketogenic diets in mental and brain disorders, evidence suggests that it is effective in schizophrenic patients.

6. Longer life

Currently, evidence suggests that high-fat and low-carbohydrate diets such as the ketogenic diet lead to longer shelf life than low-fat diets. A large study of more than 1 adult in 5 countries found that high carbohydrate consumption was associated with higher death risk, but lower healthy fat intake decreased death risk.

In fact, saturated fat consumption has an inverse relationship with myocardial infarction, which means it protects you against the risk of a stroke!

How to lose weight effectively with keto diet

The exact ratio recommended for daily intake of macronutrients - fat, carbohydrates, and protein - varies depending on your goal and your health. Your current age, gender, mobility, and body composition are important in determining the amount of carbohydrate and fat you consume.

In the traditional ketogenic diet, the total amount of carbohydrate intake was limited to 1 to 2 grams daily. The total amount of carbohydrate intake is the net carbohydrate intake after subtracting the fiber. Because fiber is not digestible it cannot be considered as carbohydrate intake.

In a restricted ketogenic diet, about 2 to 4 per cent of calories come from fat, about 2 to 3 per cent from proteins and about 2 per cent from carbohydrates. But in a more balanced keto diet, you have more flexibility.

HOW DO I PREPARE FOR MY KETO DIET?

So far we have explained the function of the ketogenic diet and you are familiar with this diet, but how to start a ketogenic diet? Although there are many different ways you can try to start the keto, the best results usually come from the following five steps:

- Step 1: Quickly cut glucose from carbohydrate foods, including grains, starchy vegetables, fruits, and others;

- Step Two: This pushes you to find an alternative source of fuel: fat (avocado, coconut oil, salmon).

- Stage Three: Without glucose the body also starts to burn fat and produce ketones.

- Step Four: When the ketone level in the blood reaches a certain point, you get into ketosis.

- Stage Five: This high ketone level can cause fast and steady weight loss until you reach healthy and stable body weight.

Here I have prepared the list of what should we eat and what we shouldn't!

Here's a list of foods you should limit or eliminate in a ketogenic diet:

- Sugar Foods: Soda, Juice, Smoothie, Cake, Ice Cream, Chocolate and more.

- Cereals and starches: Products based on flour, rice, pasta, cereals and more.

- Fruit: All fruits except a small number of berries such as strawberries.

- Beans and Beans: Peas, Red Beans, Lentils, Peas and more.

- Roots and cuttings: potatoes, carrots and more.

- Some seasonings and sauces: These are often those that contain unhealthy sugars or fats.

- Unhealthy fats: Limit processed vegetable oil and mayonnaise and the like.

- Alcohol: Due to its high carbohydrate content, it does not allow you to enter the ketosis phase.

- Sugar-free foods: These foods often contain high sugar alcohols, which in some cases affect the surface of ketones, these kinds of foods are usually processed at a high level

And if you are on a ketogenic diet you should use the following foods to base your diet on:

1. Meat: Veal, mutton, beef, chicken, and turkey.

2. Oily Fish: Salmon, Salmon, and Mackerel.

3. Eggs: It is best to use eggs that are enriched with omega-3s.

4. Butter and cream: Use as many animal products you can.

5. Cheese: Unprocessed cheese such as cream cheese, goat cheese, cheddar cheese, blue cheese or mozzarella.

6. Nuts and seeds: almonds, walnuts, flax seeds, pumpkin seeds, chia seeds and so on.

7. Healthy Oils: Set your preference for using olive oil, coconut oil, and avocado oil.

8. Avocado

9. Low Carb Vegetables: Mostly green vegetables, tomatoes, onions, chilli peppers and more.

10. Seasonings: You can use pepper salt, a variety of herbs and spices.

It is better to build your diet often on whole foods.

Here are some tips to improve your ketogenic diet:

1. Do not load up on protein

The difference between a ketogenic diet and other low-carbohydrate diets is in not loading up the protein. Fat-like proteins aren't an essential part of the ketogenic diet. Our body is able to convert protein into glucose which means that if you eat a lot of protein you will have a harder time getting into the ketosis phase.

2. Keep track of your macronutrients

Macronutrients are pure fat, protein, and carbohydrates. For this reason, we recommend installing macronutrient counters to know the exact amount of these ingredients.

3. Use ketogenic supplements for a better answer

The use of common keto supplements can faster the results and remain in ketosis. Additionally, take the leucine amino acid supplement as it breaks directly into acetyl-CoA. It is one of the body's most important ketogenic amino acids. While other amino acids are converted to glucose, ketones may be generated using acetyl-CoA. Cottage cheese and eggs contain this amino acid.

4. Drink water

It's very important to drink lots of water. Drinking enough water will prevent you from feeling tired and vital for digestion and hunger suppression. Seek to have 2 glasses of water every day.

5. Don't cheat

Finally, don't have a day of cheating on the ketogenic diet, but why? Because a cheat day meal contains high carbohydrates. By consuming carbohydrates, you exit the ketosis phase and return to the first point.

But if you can't resist cheating, you may have the side effects of starting a ketogenic diet again. But because you are already in the ketosis phase, you will be able to return to this phase more quickly.

FASTING IN A KETOGENIC DIET

It is safe for most people to have a fasting or ketogenic diet at the same time. However, pregnant women, breastfeeding mothers, and people with eating disorders should avoid fasting.

People with heart disease or diabetes should also consult a physician before combining a keto diet with fasting. Although this is useful, it may not be suitable for everyone.

It can be said that by fasting in the ketogenic diet you will be able to enter the ketosis phase faster and also burn more fat.

TIPS FOR KETO-DIETS OUTSIDE THE HOUSE

When you eat outside, having a ketogenic diet will not be difficult. Most restaurants serve you with all kinds of meat and fish. So when you go to the restaurant, choose from the meat menu and replace the high carbohydrate foods with vegetables.

An egg meal is also a great choice, for example, you can order egg or meat omelettes. Another tasty choice is a breadless hamburger and substitutes fried potatoes for vegetables.

GETTING OUT OF THE KETOGENIC DIET

To quit the keto diet but still keep your weight constant, just do the following:

Increase Carbohydrate Consumption: You have stubbornly counted carbohydrates. Now you don't need to count carbohydrates accurately to get out of the ketogenic diet. Increase your carbohydrate intake gradually. Continue to add carbohydrates one meal or snack at a time until you are enjoying them safely throughout the day.

Consume more protein: Consider adding lean protein such as chicken breast, fish, meat, eggs. Protein increases the heat effect and helps you burn more calories.

To get out of the ketogenic diet while maintaining your weight, provide 2 percent of calories with protein, 2 percent with fat, and the rest with healthy fats.

Side effects of the ketogenic diet and how to minimize it:

Although the ketogenic diet is safe for healthy people, it can lead to early side effects while your body is consistent.

This is often known as the keto flu and usually ends within a few days.

Keto influenza includes poor energy and mental function, increased hunger, sleeping disorders, nausea, gastrointestinal distress, and decreased sports performance.

To minimize these, you can try a typical low-carb diet during the first few weeks. This allows you to remind your body that it can burn its fats before you completely eliminate all carbohydrates.

A ketogenic diet can also alter the balance of water and minerals in your body, so adding salt to your meals or taking mineral supplements can be a good help.

For minerals, try to get between 3000 and 4000 mg of sodium, 1000 mg of potassium, and 300 mg of magnesium per day to minimize side effects.

At least initially, it is important to eat to be full and avoid excess calories. Usually, a ketogenic diet will reduce weight without calorie restriction.

LAST WORD...

The ketogenic diet is great for people who are overweight, diabetics, and those who want to improve their metabolic health. But this diet may not be suitable for professional athletes and those who want to increase their muscle mass and weight. Like all diets and all kinds of weight loss, a ketogenic diet can only be effective if you are steadfast in following it and following it for a long time.

RECIPES

RECIPES

BREAKFAST

BREAKFAST

KETO COCONUT PORRIDGE

Servings: 1 cup | Total Time: 10 minutes

Nutrition Information

Calories: 486| Carbs: 4 grams | Fats: 49 grams

INGREDIENTS:

- ◆ 1 Largeegg, beaten
- ◆ 1tablespoon/8gcoconut flour
- ◆ 1 pinch/0.2gground psyllium husk powder
- ◆ 1 pinch/0.36g salt
- ◆ 1 ounce /30gbutter or coconut oil

INSTRUCTIONS:

1. Combine the egg coconut flour, psyllium husk powder and salt in a medium bowl and mix.

2. Melt butter and the coconut cream over low heat. Gradually stir in the egg mixture, combine until you achieve a creamy and thick texture.

3. Serve your dish with cream or coconut milk. use fresh or frozen berries for the topping and enjoy!

KETO MUSHROOM OMELETTE

Servings: 1 cup | Total Time: 15 minutes

Nutrition Information

Calories: 517| Carbs: 5 grams | Fats: 44 grams

INGREDIENTS:

- ◆ ¼ yellow onion, chopped
- ◆ 3 Large eggs
- ◆ 4 large mushrooms, sliced
- ◆ 1 ounce /30g butter, for frying
- ◆ 1 ounce /30g (60ml) shredded cheese
- ◆ salt and pepper to taste

INSTRUCTIONS:

1. Crack the eggs and pour them into a mixing bowl with a pinch of salt and pepper. Whisk the eggs with a fork until the texture is smooth and sparkling.

2. Melt the butter over medium heat, in a frying pan. Add the mushrooms and onion to the saucepan, stirring until tender texture, then pour in the egg mixture, surrounded by the veggies.

3. Sprinkle cheese over the egg as the omelette starts to cook and become firm but still has a little raw egg on top.

4. Using a spatula, ease carefully around the omelette's sides, then fold it over in half. Lift the pan from the heat when it starts turning golden brown underneath and slip the omelette on to a tray.

ICED TEA

Servings: 1 cup | Total Time: 10 minutes + 2 hours

INGREDIENTS:

- ◆ 1 cup/225ml cold water
- ◆ ½ tea bag
- ◆ ½ cup/125ml ice cubes
- ◆ Flavourings can be your choice, such as fresh mint

INSTRUCTIONS:

1. Mix in a pitcher the tea, flavouring and half of the cold water and leave in the fridge for 1-2 hours until it becomes adequately cold.

2. Remove the flavouring and teabag and substitute them with the same or new flavouring as your preference.

3. Add cold water and serve with ice cubes.

MCGRIDDLE CASSEROLE

Servings: 1 | Total Time: 15 minutes

Nutrition Information

Calories: 447.63| Carbs: 2.87 grams | Fats: 36.04 grams

INGREDIENTS:

- 1/4 cup/186g of flaxseed
- A cup/96g of almond flour
- ½ teaspoon/1.17 g of onion powder
- 1 pound/about 2.5 g sausage
- ¼ teaspoon/0.17g of sage
- Large egg
- 1 tablespoon/20g of Maple Syrup
- 4 tablespoon/56.5 of butter, melted
- ½ teaspoon/1.64g garlic powder
- 1 ounce/about 2 g cheddar cheese
- Salt and pepper in the required amount

INSTRUCTIONS:

1. preheat to 350 degrees Fahrenheit. Place a pot on the stove over medium heat, then sausage and some butter, stir in a wooden spoon and keep getting brownish. In a separate bowl, add all the dry ingredients and then the wet ingredients.

2. Just keep for 2 tablespoons of maple syrup for later. Combine all in properly. Add the cheese to the mix and stir again. Remove all the remaining ingredients (including the rest of the butter) after the sausage has browned and slightly crispy and combine well.

3. Prepare a plate. Pour the Castrol mixture over it. Add 2 tablespoons of the remaining syrup. You can use a bigger bowl if you want to make the Castrol thicker. In this situation, you can also reduce the cooking time.

4. Place the pan in the oven and wait 45-55 minutes until it is fully cooked. Take from the oven after baking and allow to cool. Remove the paper by raising the edges of the skin. Cut and serve.

WAFFLE AND CHEDDAR

Servings: 12 | Total Time: 15 minutes

Nutrition Information

Calories: 195.5| Carbs: 3.49 grams | Fats: 17.47 grams

INGREDIENTS:

- 1 teaspoon/1g dried common sage
- ½ teaspoon/3.2g of salt
- 3 tablespoon/39g of coconut oil, melted
- 1/3 cups/41g of coconut flour
- ¼ teaspoon/0.82g of garlic powder
- 2 cup/456g of canned coconut milk
- Half a cup/113g of water
- 3 teaspoon/12g baking powder
- Large egg
- 1 cup/125g of cheddar cheese, chopped

INSTRUCTIONS:

1. Preheat a medium-heat waffle maker, according to the manufacturer's instructions.

2. Mix the baking powder and the seasonings in a bowl of flour.

3. Add the liquid and stir to form a firm paste.

4. Add the cheese to the mixture.

5. Grease the top and bottom pages of the waffle maker and then spread one-third of the dough with a spoon on the surface.

6. Fasten the lid and continue to cook until the steam rises from the machine and the top plate opens freely without adhering to the waffle.

BUTTERMILK FLUFFY PANCAKES

Servings: 1 | Total Time: 15 minutes

Nutrition Information

Calories: 422| Carbs: 13 grams | Fats: 19.28 grams

INGREDIENTS:

- 2 large eggs, separated yellow and white part of the egg
- 4 white part of the egg
- ½ cup/120g of buttermilk
- 1 teaspoon/4.2g vanilla extract
- 1 tablespoon/25g of protein powder
- ¼ cup/28g of coconut flour
- 1 teaspoon/4g baking powder
- ¼ tablespoon/2g of cinnamon
- 1 Pack of Stevia
- Butter or oil in the required amount

INSTRUCTIONS:

1. Pour a little salt into the whites of the egg (which you have separated from the yolks), stirring using a mixer.

2. Mix the buttermilk, egg yolk, extra egg whites and vanilla extract into a bowl.

3. Mix the coconut flour, protein powder, baking powder, and cinnamon in a separate bowl.

4. Add dry ingredients to moist ingredients and blend together

5. Grease the pan with butter. Bring a quarter cup of dough into the saucepan and shake slightly to spread the dough.

6. When one side is baked, turn to make the other side golden brown.

VEGGIE KETO SCRAMBLE

Servings: 1 | Total Time: 20 minutes

Nutrition Information

Calories: 415| Carbs: 4 grams | Fats: 31 grams

INGREDIENTS:

- 1 tablespoon/14g of butter
- 1 ounce /30g parmesan cheese, shredded
- 1 ounce/30g mushroom, sliced
- 1 ounce /30g red bell peppers, diced
- 3 large eggs
- ½ scallion, chopped
- salt and ground black pepper

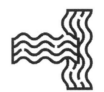

INSTRUCTIONS:

1. Heat the butter over medium heat, in a large frying pan.

2. Add the sliced mushrooms, chopped red peppers, salt and fry until smooth.

3. Crack the eggs into the saucepan and quickly stir it until all is well incorporated.

4. Move the spatula across the skillet's bottom and side on form large, soft curds. Cook until the egg is clear, but the eggs are not dry. Put the scramble on a plate with shredded parmesan and scallions to top.

KETO SEAFOOD OMELETTE

Servings: 2 | Total Time: 20 minutes

Nutrition Information

Calories: 872| Carbs: 4 grams | Fats: 83 grams

INGREDIENTS:

- 5 ounce/150g cooked shrimp or seafood mix
- 1 tablespoon fresh chives or dried chives
- 6 large eggs
- 1 red chilli pepper
- ½ tablespoon/ fennel seeds or ground cumin
- 2 garlic cloves (optional)
- 2 tablespoon/26g of olive oil
- salt and pepper to taste
- ½ cup/125ml of mayonnaise

INSTRUCTIONS:

1. Have the broiler preheated. Broil the shrimp or fish together with minced garlic, chili, fennel seeds, cumin, salt, and pepper in olive oil. Set aside and let cool to the temperature of the room. To the cooled seafood mixture, apply mayonnaise and chives.

2. Whisk up the eggs. Top with pepper and salt. With plenty of butter or oil, fry in a non-stick frying dish. Once the omelette is almost prepared, add the seafood mixture. Fold it, lower the heat, and allow to set fully.

KETO BREAKFAST SANDWICH

Servings: 2 | Total Time: 15 minutes

Nutrition Information

Calories: 354| Carbs: 4 grams | Fats: 30 grams

INGREDIENTS:

- ◆ 2 tablespoon of butter
- ◆ 1 ounce/30g smoked deli ham
- ◆ a few drops of tabasco or Worcestershire sauce(optional)
- ◆ 4 large eggs
- ◆ salt and pepper
- ◆ 2 ounce/50g of cheddar cheese or Edam cheese, slices

INSTRUCTIONS:

1. Melt the butter, mix in the remaining bread ingredients, and microwave for 90 seconds. Let the bread slightly cool, then slice it into two slices.

2. Grease a nonstick skillet or frying pan, heat it, and use it for cooking the egg and toasting the bread slices.

3. 3. Assemble the sandwich, a slice of bread, overlapped with cheese, ham, bacon, and then the bread slice.

KETO BLT WITH CLOUD BREAD

Servings: 2 | Total Time: 45 minutes

Nutrition Information

Calories: 800| Carbs: 7 grams | Fats:75 grams

INGREDIENTS:

- ◆ 3 Large eggs
- ◆ ¼ teaspoon cream of tartar (optional)
- ◆ ½ tablespoon/4g of ground psyllium husk powder
- ◆ 1pinch/0.36 of salt
- ◆ 4 tablespoon/58g of mayonnaise
- ◆ 5 ounces/150g of bacon
- ◆ 4 ounces/110g cream cheese
- ◆ 2 ounces/50g of lettuce
- ◆ ½ teaspoon/2.5g baking powder
- ◆ 1 tomato, thinly sliced

INSTRUCTIONS:

1. Preheat oven to 300 degrees F.

2. Separate the eggs, with egg whites in one bowl and egg yolks in another. It is better to serve the egg whites, Unlike plastic, in a metal or ceramic bowl

3. Whip egg whites with salt (and tartar cream) until very firm, better use an electric mixer. You need to be able to shift the bowl over without the egg whites moving

4. Add and blend cream cheese, psyllium husk, and baking powder.

5. Fold the egg whites slowly into the egg yolk mixture-try to keep the egg whites in the air

6. Place two dollops of the mixture on a baking tray covered with paper. Stretch the circles up to 1/2 inch (1 cm) thick parts with a spatula.

7. Bake for about 25 minutes in the middle of the oven before they transform to golden colour.

KETO SCRAMBLED EGGS WITH HALLOUMI CHEESE

Servings: 2 | Total Time: 25 minutes

Nutrition Information

Calories: 657| Carbs: 4 grams | Fats:59 grams

INGREDIENTS:

- 3 ounces/75g halloumi cheese, diced
- 2 tablespoon olive oil
- 4 tablespoon fresh parsley, chopped
- 2 scallions, chopped
- 4 ounces/110g bacon, diced
- 4 large eggs
- salt and pepper to taste
- 2 ounces/50g pitted olives

INSTRUCTIONS:

1. Heat olive oil in a frying pan and fry halloumi to a medium degree, scallions and bacon until golden.

2. Whisk them all in a small bowl along with the parsley, eggs, salt, and pepper.

3. Pour the egg mixture over the bacon and cheese into the frying saucepan.

4. Reduce the heat, add the olives and then mix for a few minutes.

KETO EGGS ON THE GO

Servings: 4 | Total Time: 25 minutes

Nutrition Information

Calories: 205| Carbs: 1 grams | Fats: 16 grams

INGREDIENTS:

- ◆ 8 large eggs
- ◆ salt and pepper to taste
- ◆ 2/3 ounces/75g cooked bacon

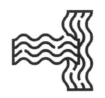

INSTRUCTIONS:

1. The oven should be preheated to 400 ° F.

2. Place the liners for a cupcake. Be mindful that even non-stick surfaces can be easily adhered to by eggs except for silicon varieties.

3. Crack one egg in each form and add season filling to taste.

4. Bake for about 15 minutes in the oven, or until the eggs are cooked.

KETO WESTERN OMELETTE

Servings: 2 | Total Time: 30 minutes

Nutrition Information

Calories: 687| Carbs: 6 grams | Fats: 56 grams

INGREDIENTS:

- 6 eggs
- 5 ounces/155g smoked deli ham, diced
- 2 tablespoon heavy whipping cream or sour cream
- ½ yellow onion, finely chopped
- salt and pepper
- ½ green bell pepper, finely chopped
- 3 ounces/75g(150ml) shredded cheese, divided
- 2 ounces/50g butter

INSTRUCTIONS:

1. Whisk eggs and cream in a mixing bowl, until the structure is smooth, then add salt and pepper.

2. Add half the shredded cheese and blend well.

3. Melt the butter over medium heat, in a large frying pan.

4. Fry the diced ham a few minutes in butter, onion and peppers. Add the egg mixture and fry until almost firm on the omelette. Be careful not to make the edges burn.

5. Reduce the heat after a while. Sprinkle the remaining cheese on top and fold the omelette if you wish. It should be served instantly, and the omelette should be cut in half.

SCRAMBLED EGGS WITH BASIL AND BUTTER

Servings: 1 | Total Time: 10 minutes

Nutrition Information

Calories: 641| Carbs: 3 grams | Fats: 59 grams

INGREDIENTS:

♦ 2 tablespoon butter

♦ 2 tablespoon fresh basil

♦ 2 tablespoon heavy whipping cream

♦ 2 ounces/50g(100ml) shredded cheesc

♦ 2 large eggs

♦ salt and ground black pepper

INSTRUCTIONS:

1. 1. Melt butter over low heat in a saucepan.

2. Add cracked eggs, cheese, cream and seasoning to a small bowl. Stir with a light movement and add to the pan.

3. Stir with a spatula from edge site to centre until the eggs are scrambled. stir on low heat if you prefer it creamy or soft.

4. design topping with fresh basil.

KETO PANCAKES WITH BERRIES AND WHIPPED CREAM

Servings: 4 | Total Time: 25 minutes

Nutrition Information

Calories: 424| Carbs: 4 grams | Fats: 39 grams

INGREDIENTS:

- ◆ 4 large eggs
- ◆ 2 ounces/50g fresh raspberries or fresh blueberries or fresh strawberries
- ◆ 7 ounces/200g (225ml) cottage cheese
- ◆ 1 tablespoon/8g ground psyllium husk powder
- ◆ 2 ounces/50g butter or coconut oil
- ◆ 1 cup/225ml heavy whipping cream

INSTRUCTIONS:

1. In a medium-sized cup, add the eggs, cottage cheese and psyllium husk and blend together. Let them thicken up a little for 5-10 minutes.

2. Warm-up a non-stick skillet with butter or oil. Fry each side of the pancakes at medium-low heat for 3–4 minutes. Don't make them too large, after all, they are going to be difficult to flip.

3. Add cream and whip until soft peaks shape in a separate bowl.

4. Eat the pancakes with your favourite whipped cream and berries.

LUNCH

FISH STEW

Servings: 4 | Total Time: 25 minutes

Nutrition Information

Calories: 424| Carbs: 4 grams | Fats: 39 grams

INGREDIENTS:

- 2 cups coconut milk or milk
- 1 tablespoon lemon juice
- 450 g milkfish or tilapia
- ½ cup ground chopped coriander
- 1small onion
- 3 cups vegetable juice
- Salt and pepper to taste
- 1 pc of red chilli pepper
- 1 number of Jalapeño pepper

INSTRUCTIONS:

1. Pour coconut milk and vegetable juice into the pot and boil.

2. Chop the Bell peppers and onions.

3. separate the Jalapeño pepper seeds and chop it.

4. Remove the fish blades and cut them into square pieces.

5. Put the Bell peppers, onion and Jalapeño pepper in the pot filled with water and boil for about 15 minutes.

6. Add salt, pepper and fish pieces and allow the ingredients to boil for another 5 minutes until the fish is cooked to the full. Attach the coriander and lemon juice and serve

KETO PIZZA

Servings: 2 | Total Time: 25 minutes

Nutrition Information

Calories: 1043| Carbs: 5 grams | Fats: 90 grams

INGREDIENTS:

Crust

- ♦ 4 eggs
- ♦ 6 oz/175g(375ml) shredded cheese, preferably mozzarella or provolone

Topping

- ♦ 1 tablespoon dried oregano
- ♦ 3 tablespoon unsweetened tomato sauce
- ♦ 5 oz./150g(325ml) shredded cheese
- ♦ 1½ oz./40g pepperoni
- ♦ olives (optional)

For serving

- ♦ 4 tablespoon olive oil
- ♦ 2 oz./55g leafy greens
- ♦ sea salt and ground black pepper

INSTRUCTIONS:

1. Oven preheated to 200 ° C (400 ° F). First Start with crust making. Crack eggs into a bowl of medium size, and add shredded cheese. Stir it all up until it combines nicely.

2. Use a spatula on a baking sheet lined with parchment paper to spread the cheese and egg batter. You may form two circles of pizza or just shape one large rectangular pizza. Let them stay in the oven for 15 minutes until the pizza crust becomes golden brown .Remove and allow to cool for 3 minutes.

3. Turn up the oven to 450 ° F (225 ° C). Pour the tomato sauce over the crust, then sprinkle with the oregano on top. Fill with cheese, pepperoni and olives Bake for an additional 5-10 minutes or until the pizza turns golden brown. Serve with a simple side salad.

KETO HAMBURGER PATTIES WITH CREAMY TOMATO SAUCE AND FRIED CABBAGE

Servings: 4 | Total Time: 60 minutes

Nutrition Information

Calories: 923| Carbs: 10 grams | Fats: 78 grams

INGREDIENTS:

Hamburger patties

- 1½ lbs/650g ground beef
- 3 oz./80g crumbled feta cheese
- 1 egg
- 1 tablespoon olive oil, for frying
- 1 teaspoon salt
- ¼ teaspoon ground black pepper
- 2 oz./50g fresh parsley, finely chopped
- 2 tablespoon butter, for frying

Gravy

- 2 tablespoon tomato paste or ajvar relish
- ¾ cup/175ml heavy whipping cream
- 1 oz./30g fresh parsley, coarsely chopped
- salt and pepper to taste

Fried cabbage

- 4½ oz./125g butter
- salt and pepper
- 1½ lbs/650g shredded green cabbage

INSTRUCTIONS:

Gravy and hamburger patties

1. Add all the ingredients to a large bowl for the hamburgers. Mix it with a wooden spoon or with your clean hands. Be mindful that when you mix it, it can be tough you Need your wet hands to shape eight oblong patties.

2. Add the butter and olive oil over medium-high heat to a large frying pan until the patties turn a nice colour. Flip them whilst cooking a few times.

3. Whisk the tomato paste and cream together in a small bowl. Add this mixture to the pan when the patties are nearly done. Remove and let simmer for a few minutes. Garnish with salt and pepper. Sprinkle on top with chopped parsley before serving.

Fried cabbage

1. Using a food processor or sharp knife finely cut the cabbage.

2. To a large frying pan, add butter.

3. Place the saucepan over medium-high heat and fry the shredded cabbage for at least 15 minutes or until it turns golden brown and wilts around the edges.

4. Regularly stir and reduce heat to the bottom.

5. Season with salt and pepper.

KETO LASAGNA

Servings: 6 | Total Time: 80 minutes

Nutrition Information

Calories: 873| Carbs: 9 grams | Fats: 74 grams

INGREDIENTS:

Lasagna sheets

- 10 oz./27g cream cheese
- 1 teaspoon salt
- 8 eggs, beaten
- 5 tablespoon/40g ground psyllium husk powder

Cheese topping

- 2 cups/475ml crème fraîche or sour cream
- 2 oz./50g parmesan cheese, grated
- ½ cup/125ml fresh parsley, chopped
- 5 oz./155g mozzarella cheese, shredded
- ½ teaspoon salt
- ¼ teaspoon ground black pepper

Meat sauce

- 1¼ lbs/550g ground beef
- 2 tablespoon olive oil
- 1 yellow onion, chopped
- ½ cup/125ml of water
- 1 garlic clove,chopped
- 3 tablespoon tomato paste

- ½ tablespoon dried basil
- 1 tablespoon salt
- ¼ teaspoon ground black pepper

INSTRUCTIONS:

Lasagna sheets

1. Preheat oven to 300 ° F (150 ° C). Line a sheet of parchment paper for baking.

2. Whisk the eggs, cream cheese and salt in a medium-sized bowl once they become smooth. whisk in the husk of the psyllium, then set aside for a few minutes.

3. Apply the batter to the parchment paper centre then place another baking paper on top.

4. Bake for about 10-12 minutes each sheet with a parchment paper.

5. Set to cool off. Remove the paper and slice the pasta into meal-fitting sheets.

Meat sauce

1. Heat the olive oil in a large saucepan over medium-high heat. Add the onion and garlic, stirring until smooth. Next add the beef, tomato paste and spices and then mix thoroughly until the beef is no longer pink in colour.

2. Add water to the paste, bring to a boil, then reduce heat and allow to simmer for at least 15 minutes or until most water evaporates Because these lasagna sheets do not soak up as much liquid as typical sheets, the sauce should be on the drier side.

3. Preheat the oven to 400 ° F (200 ° C). Grease the dish.

Cheese topping

1. Mix mozzarella cheese with sour cream and parmesan cheese at 80 per cent. save two parmesan cheese spoons for the last topping. Add salt and pepper, then stir.

2. Alternatively, in the baking dish, layer the pasta sheets and meat sauce, starting with the pasta, accompanied by the meat sauce.

3. Place the cheese mixture over the spaghetti, and finish with the parmesan cheese.

4. Bake in the oven for about 30 minutes, or until the top of the lasagna is nicely brown Serve with your preferred dressing and a green salad.

KETO STEAK WITH BÉARNAISE SAUCE

Servings: 4 | Total Time: 25 minutes

Nutrition Information

Calories: 1124| Carbs: 3 grams | Fats: 103 grams

INGREDIENTS:

Béarnaise sauce

- 2 tablespoon fresh tarragon, finely chopped
- 4rib-eye steaks, at room temperature
- 4 egg yolks, at room temperature
- 2 teaspoon white wine vinegar
- ½ teaspoon onion powder
- 10 oz.butter
- salt and pepper
- 2 tablespoon/275g butter
- salt and pepper to taste

Salad

- 2 oz./50g lettuce
- 8 oz./225g cherry tomatoes, quartered
- 2 oz./50g arugula lettuce

INSTRUCTIONS:

We will start with the sauce!

1. Separate the yolks and whites of the eggs and place the yolks in a small bowl which is heat-resistance. (Save the whites later). In another small bowl, stir the vinegar, tarragon and onion powder together. Whisk the yolks until smooth, using a hand mixer.

2. Melt the butter gently in a microwave oven for saucepan or. Don't let it get too hot; without getting burnt, you should be able to put your finger in it.

3. Carefully add the butter into the yolks while continuing whisking. Increase speed as the sauce begins thickening. The white milk protein produced at the bottom of the melted butter should not be added into the sauce.

4. Whisk in the spices and vinegar. Season with salt and pepper. Make sure you keep the sauce warm

5. Grill the meat to your personal taste. Serve with the salad and béarnaise sauce .

KETO ZOODLES BOLOGNESE

Servings: 6 | Total Time: 50 minutes

Nutrition Information

Calories: 425| Carbs: 10 grams | Fats: 31 grams

INGREDIENTS:

- 1 yellow onion
- 1 tablespoon Worcestershire sauce
- 3 oz./75g celery stalks
- 1½ lbs/650g ground beef
- 3 oz./75g butter or olive oil
- 2 tablespoon tomato paste
- 1 garlic clove
- 14 oz./400g crushed tomatoes
- ¼ teaspoon pepper
- 1 tablespoon dried oregano or dried basil
- 1teaspoon salt
- water

Zoodles

- 2 tablespoon butter or olive oil
- 2 lbs/900g zucchini
- salt or pepper to taste

INSTRUCTIONS:

1. Chop the vegetables. Stir in butter or olive oil and add the ground beef until tender. Sauté on high heat until all has turned into a nice colour. Add remaining ingredients, stir on medium-high for 15 minutes.

2. Lower the heat a little bit more. If the sauce becomes too thick, add water. Let it cook for 20 or more. Clearly, the more the sauce allowed to simmer the taste will be greater.

3. Meanwhile, do the noodles. To make thin stripes of zucchini use a peeler. Heat a frying pan and quickly toss them into butter or olive oil for not more than a minute.

4. after tasting, you can add more salt and pepper.

5. Serve the hot sauce on top of the warm noodles. Finish off with a good parmesan cheese grating.

Hint: if you want to limit carbs, you can skip the tomato paste!

LOW-CARB EGGPLANT PIZZA

Servings: 4 | Total Time: 55 minutes

Nutrition Information

Calories: 671| Carbs: 13 grams | Fats: 50 grams

INGREDIENTS:

- ◆ 2 eggplant
- ◆ 1 onion
- ◆ 1/3 cup/75ml olive oil, for brushing and frying
- ◆ 2 garlic cloves
- ◆ ½ teaspoon cinnamon (optional)
- ◆ ¾ lb/325g ground beef
- ◆ ¾ cup/175ml tomato sauce
- ◆ 1 teaspoon salt
- ◆ ½ teaspoon pepper
- ◆ 10 oz./275g(600ml) shredded cheese
- ◆ ¼ cup/60ml chopped fresh oregano

INSTRUCTIONS:

1. After Preheating the oven to 400 ° F (200 ° C). then Cut the eggplants one centimetre thick. Coat on both sides with olive oil, and put on a baking sheet lined with parchment paper. Bake for about twenty minutes or until light brown.

2. Fry the garlic and onion for about 3-4 minutes in remaining olive oil until softened. Add the beef and sauté until well done. Stir in tomato sauce and season with salt and pepper. Let it simmer for 10 minutes or until warm.

3. Take the slices of eggplant from the oven and spread the meat mixture over the top. Sprinkle with Oregano and Cheese. Put in the oven for about 10 minutes or until you have the cheese melted.

4. Serve with olive oil and a green salad.

GRILLED FISH

Servings: 4 | Total Time: 40 minutes

Nutrition Information

Calories: 300| Carbs: 3 grams | Fats: 21 grams

INGREDIENTS:

- ♦ 1 lemon
- ♦ ½ Chopped coriander
- ♦ 3 Garlic cubes
- ♦ ½ Jalapeño pepper
- ♦ ½ teaspoon black pepper
- ♦ ½ teaspoon salt
- ♦ ¼ cup olive oil
- ♦ 500 grams of salmon fillet

INSTRUCTIONS:

1. Grate lemon peel and chop garlic.

2. To make the sauce, add garlic, lemon peel, Jalapeño pepper, coriander, salt, pepper and olive oil in a pan.

3. Peel the skin of the fish and cut into relatively large cubic pieces.

4. Soak the fish in the sauce and set the fish for 20 minutes.

5. Grill the fish and place on a grill or grill plate and rotate it for about 4 minutes to the other side.

6. Serve it!

Hint: If you use wooden skewers, be sure to put them in the water for 1 hour before using them until they are exposed to fire, but if skewers are iron you do not need to!

KETO LEMON CHICKEN

Servings: 4 | Total Time: 40 minutes

Nutrition Information

Calories: 390| Carbs: 11 grams | Fats: 18 grams

INGREDIENTS:

- ◆ 1kg Grilled Chicken with Bones
- ◆ ¼ cup of soy sauce
- ◆ 3 tablespoons onion, chopped
- ◆ 2 tablespoons olive oil
- ◆ 1 tablespoon salt
- ◆ 2 Garlic
- ◆ 2 lemons
- ◆ 1 orange
- ◆ ½cup Chopped parsley

INSTRUCTIONS:

1. 1. Cut the onions and garlic.

2. Grate the orange peel. Approximately a teaspoon of grated orange peel is needed.

3. Take the orange juice. Around one-fourth of an orange juice is needed.

4. Grate lemon peel. A teaspoon of grated lemon peel is needed.

5. Take lemon juice. You need about a quarter cup of lemon juice.

6. Pour Parsley, onion, orange peel, orange juice, lemon peel, lemon juice, garlic, olive oil, soy sauce and salt in the mixer and mix them.

7. Put a quarter cup of the blended mixture aside and put the rest of the ingredients in a zippered plastic bag with the chicken. With the chickens, they should be kept in the bag for 2 hours.

8. After 2 hours, remove the chicken from the bag and place it on a grill pan to roast. It takes about 15 minutes to grill the chicken.

9. After the chickens are fully cooked and roasted, pour the rest of the sauce which you had been prepared on the chicken surface and serve.

HOMEMADE SAUSAGES

Servings: 4 | Total Time: 40 minutes

Nutrition Information

Calories: 319| Carbs: 2 grams | Fats: 20 grams

INGREDIENTS:

- 450 grams of veal (or lamb)
- 3 teaspoons paprika
- 2 teaspoons crushed garlic
- ½ teaspoon of fennel (or coriander seeds)
- 1 teaspoon salt
- ¼ teaspoon red pepper
- ½ teaspoon black pepper
- ¼ teaspoon cumin
- ¼ teaspoon cinnamon
- Fresh parsley
- Sausage casing

INSTRUCTIONS:

1. Chop the meat.

2. Add the spices to the meat and mix. Then cover the plate surface and place for 2 hours in the freezer.

3. When you have removed the meat from the freezer, grind it with the meat grinder and mix it again by hand or with a mixer until the spices are thoroughly mixed with the meat.

4. Attach the sausage head to the meat grinder. Pull the sausage pod to the bottom.

5. Pour the meat into the meat grinder to come out of the sausage head and into the Sausage casing. Try to squeeze the meat completely.

6. Tie the end of the Sausage casing. Cut the meat inside the Sausage casing as desired and by hand, and wrap the meat in it to form a sausage.

7. Finally, if you see air inside the sheath, pierce the sheath with a needle to let the air out.

8. The sausages are ready. You can store these sausages in the freezer or use them right now.

Tips on preparing sausages

9. Because of the different types of sausages, the spices used are quite varied. You can customize or add these spices to your taste and family, or even change them to your liking.

10. Try not to store sausages in the freezer for more than 2 months and eat them for less than 2 months.

11. Remember, these sausages may not taste exactly like the factory sausages! But they are tasty and healthier.

KETO LOW CARB SANDWICH LUNCHBOX

Servings: 4 | Total Time: 25 minutes

Nutrition Information

Calories: 569| Carbs: 15 grams | Fats: 56 grams

INGREDIENTS:

- 12 Slices Genoa Salami
- 12 Slices Ham
- 12 Slices Pepperoni
- 12 Provolone Slices
- 6 tablespoon Mayonnaise
- Roasted peppers
- Sliced banana peppers
- Shredded Lettuce
- about 40 black olives
- 2 apples

INSTRUCTIONS:

1. Lay ingredients and roll sandwich up. Secure the sandwich with a toothpick.

2. Place your ingredients into your Lunchbox.

3. Cover and cool it down before ready to use. Use within 3 days.

KETO MEAT PIE

Servings: 6 | Total Time: 70 minutes

Nutrition Information

Calories: 609| Carbs: 7 grams | Fats: 47 grams

INGREDIENTS:

Pie crust

- ¾ cup/100g(175ml) almond flour
- 1 pinch of salt
- 1 tablespoon/8g ground psyllium husk powder
- 4 tablespoon/35g sesame seeds
- 3 tablespoon olive oil or coconut oil, melted
- 4 tablespoon/30g coconut flour
- 1 teaspoon/5g baking powder
- 1 egg
- 4 tablespoon water

Topping

- 7 oz./200g(425ml) shredded cheese
- 8 oz./225g(250ml) cottage cheese

Filling

- ½ yellow onion, finely chopped
- 2 tablespoon butter or olive oil
- 1 tablespoon dried oregano or dried basil
- 1 garlic clove, finely chopped
- 1¼ lbs/550g ground beef or ground lamb

- salt and pepper to taste
- 4 tablespoon tomato paste or ajvar relish
- ½ cup/125ml water

INSTRUCTIONS:

1. After Preheating the oven to 350 ° F (175 ° C).

2. Fry the onion and garlic over medium heat in butter or olive oil for a few minutes, until the onion is tender. Add the ground beef and basil (or oregano). Season with salt and pepper.

3. Add the ajvar relish or tomato paste and water. Reduce the heat and allow to simmer for at minimum 20 minutes. Make the dough for the crust while the meat is simmering.

4. In a food processor, mix all the crust ingredients for a few minutes, until the dough turns into a ball. If you don't have a processor, you may mix it by hand with a fork.

5. Place a round piece of parchment paper in a well-greased panto to make removing the pie simpler when finished.

6. Layer the dough in the pan then move along the edges. Use a spatula, or fingertips well grazed. Once the crust has been shaped to the pan, make the small hole with a fork at the bottom of the crust.

7. Bake the crust 10-15 minutes beforehand. Remove from the oven and sprinkle meat into the crust. Blend together cottage cheese and shredded cheese, and layer on top of the pie.

8. Bake 30-40 minutes or more until the pie turns a golden colour.

SALADIN A JAR

Servings: 1| Total Time: 10 minutes

Nutrition Information

Calories: 875| Carbs: 11 grams | Fats: 27 grams

INGREDIENTS:

- ◆ 1 carrot
- ◆ 1 avocado
- ◆ 1 oz./30g red bell peppers
- ◆ 1 oz./30g leafy greens
- ◆ 1 oz./30g cherry tomatoes
- ◆ ½ scallion, sliced
- ◆ 4 oz./110g smoked salmon or rotisserie chicken
- ◆ ¼ cup/60ml mayonnaise or olive oil

INSTRUCTIONS:

1. Shred or chop the vegetables.

2. put the dark leafy greens at the bottom of the jar.

3. Add scallion, carrot, avocado, bell peppers and tomato in layers.

4. Top with smoked salmon or grilled chicken.

5. Add mayonnaise before serving.

KETO CAESAR SALAD

Servings: 2| Total Time: 35 minutes

Nutrition Information

Calories: 1018| Carbs: 4 grams | Fats: 87 grams

INGREDIENTS:

- salt and pepper
- 3 oz./75g bacon
- 7 oz./200g lettuce
- 1 tablespoon olive oil
- ¾ lb/235g chicken breasts
- 1 oz./30g Parmesan cheese

Dressing

- ½ lemon, zest, and juice
- ½ oz./15g Parmesan cheese, grated
- 1 garlic clove, finely chopped
- 2 tablespoon finely chopped filets of anchovies
- ½ cup/125ml mayonnaise
- salt and pepper to taste
- 1 tablespoon Dijon mustard

INSTRUCTIONS:

1. Preheat the oven to 350 ° F (175 ° C).

2. Mix the dressing ingredients with a whisk or mixer. put aside In the fridge . In a greased baking dish, put the chicken breasts.

3. Spice the chicken with salt and pepper and drizzle on top with olive oil or melted butter. Bake the chicken in the oven for about 20 minutes or until it is fully cooked through. Top if you wish. Fry the bacon until it turns crispy. Chop the lettuce and lay it on two plates as a base. Place crumbled bacon and chicken on top

4. Finish off with a good parmesan cheese grating.

KETO SALMONBURGERS WITH MASH AND LEMON BUTTER

Servings: 4| Total Time: 30 minutes

Nutrition Information

Calories: 1030| Carbs: 7 grams | Fats: 91 grams

INGREDIENTS:

Salmon burgers

- 1½ lbs/650g of salmon
- 1 egg
- ½ yellow onion
- 1 teaspoon salt
- ½ teaspoon pepper
- 2 oz./50g butter, for frying

Green mash

- 1 lb./450g broccoli
- salt and pepper to taste
- 5 oz./150g butter
- 2 oz./55g Parmesan cheese,grated

Lemon butter

- 2 tablespoon lemon juice
- 4 oz./110g butter
- salt and pepper to taste

INSTRUCTIONS:

1. Preheat the oven to 100 ° C (220 ° F). Cut the fish into small pieces and place them in a food processor, along with the rest of the burger ingredients.

2. Pulse for 30-45. Don't blend too thoroughly. It will harden the burgers. Shape 6-8 burgers and fry in enough butter or oil on each side for 4-5 minutes at medium heat. Keep them in the oven warm.

3. Cut broccoli to pieces . Whether you like, cut and slice the broccoli stem too.

4. Bring a lightly salted pot of water to a boil and add the broccoli. Cook for a couple of minutes until soft, but not until all texture is gone. And then Drain the boiling water.

5. To mix broccoli with butter and Parmesan cheese, use an immersion blender or food processor.

6. Make the lemon butter in a small bowl using electric beaters by combining the butter (at room temperature) with the lemon juice, salt and pepper.

7. Serve the sandwiches with green mash as a side and fresh lemon butter melting mass on top.

DINNER

DINNER

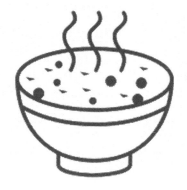

KETO CHICKEN AND FETA CHEESE PLATE

Servings: 2| Total Time: 5 minutes

Nutrition Information

Calories: 1194| Carbs: 9 grams | Fats: 102 grams

INGREDIENTS:

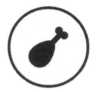

Salmon burgers

- 1½ lbs/650g of salmon
- 1 egg
- ½ yellow onion
- 1 teaspoon salt
- ½ teaspoon pepper
- 2 oz./50g butter, for frying

Green mash

- 1 lb./450g broccoli
- 5 oz./150g butter
- 2 oz./50g Parmesan cheese, grated
- salt and pepper to taste

Lemon butter

- 4 oz./110g butter
- 2 tablespoon lemon juice
- salt and pepper to taste

INSTRUCTIONS:

1. Preheat the oven to 220 ° F (100 ° C). Cut the fish into small pieces and place, along with the rest of the ingredients for the burger, in a food processor.

2. Pulse for 30-45. Don't mix too thoroughly, it can make the burgers tough.

3. Shape 6-8 burgers and fry for 4-5 minutes on each side on medium heat in enough amount of butter or oil. Keep warm in the oven.

4. Trim the broccoli and cut into small florets. Peel and chop the stem of broccoli as well if you prefer.

5. Bring a lightly salted pot of water to a boil and add the broccoli. Cook for a few minutes until soft but not until all texture is gone. Drain the boiling water.

6. Use an immersion blender or a food processor to mix the broccoli with butter and Parmesan cheese. Season and salt and pepper to taste.

7. Make the lemon butter by mixing the butter (at room temperature) with lemon juice, salt and pepper in a small bowl using electric beaters.

8. Serve the burgers with green mash as a side and a melting mass of fresh lemon butter on top.

KETO SALAMI AND BRIE CHEESE PLATE

Servings: 2| Total Time: 5 minutes

Nutrition Information

Calories: 1203| Carbs: 5 grams | Fats: 113 grams

INGREDIENTS:

- 7 oz./200g Brie cheese
- 4 oz./110g salami
- 2 oz./50g lettuce
- 1 avocado
- ½ cup/125ml macadamia nuts
- ¼ cup/60ml olive oil

INSTRUCTIONS:

1. Put cheese, salami, lettuce, avocado and nuts on a plate. Pour oil over salad and serve.

KETO ROAST BEEF AND CHEDDAR PLATE

Servings: 2| Total Time: 5 minutes

Nutrition Information

Calories: 1071| Carbs: 6 grams | Fats: 98 grams

INGREDIENTS:

- 7 oz./200g deli roast beef
- 2 tablespoon olive oil
- 5 oz./150g cheddar cheese
- 1 avocado
- salt and pepper to taste
- 1 tablespoon Dijon mustard
- 6 radishes
- 1 scallion
- ½ cup/125ml mayonnaise
- 2oz./50g lettuce

INSTRUCTIONS:

1. Place beef, cheese, avocado and radishes on a plate.

2. Add chopped onion, mustard, and mayonnaise.

3. 3. Eat with the olive oil and lettuce

ITALIAN KETO PLATE

Servings: 2| Total Time: 5 minutes

Nutrition Information

Calories: 822| Carbs: 8 grams | Fats: 40 grams

INGREDIENTS:

- 7 oz./200g mozzarella cheese
- 1/3 cup /75ml olive oil
- 2 tomatoes
- salt and pepper to taste
- 10 green olives
- 7 oz./200g prosciutto, sliced

INSTRUCTIONS:

1. Put on a plate the onions, the prosciutto, cheese and olives. Serve with olive oil and season with salt and pepper.

KETO AVOCADO, BACON AND GOAT-CHEESE SALAD

Servings: 4| Total Time: 30 minutes

Nutrition Information

Calories: 1251| Carbs: 6 grams | Fats: 123 grams

INGREDIENTS:

- ♦ 8 oz./225g goat cheese
- ♦ 4 oz./110g arugula lettuce
- ♦ 8 oz./225g bacon
- ♦ 4 oz./110g walnuts
- ♦ 2 avocados

Dressing

- ♦ salt and pepper to taste
- ♦ 2 tablespoon heavy whipping cream
- ♦ 1 tablespoon lemon juice
- ♦ ½ cup/125ml mayonnaise
- ♦ ½ cup/125ml olive oil

INSTRUCTIONS:

1. Preheat the oven to 400 degrees Fahrenheit (200 degrees Celsius) and put it on a baking large plate. Cut in half an inch (1 cm) of goat cheese and put in a baking dish. Bake the rack on the on top until golden

2. In a frying pan, fry the bacon and make them crisp.

3. Chop the avocado into pieces and coat them with Arugula. Add bacon and chicken meat. Sprinkle over the nuts.

4. For dressing Season with salt and pepper, make the sauce with lemon juice, mayonnaise, olive oil and cream using a blender.

KETO TUNA SALAD WITH BOILED EGGS

Servings: 2| Total Time: 15 minutes

Nutrition Information

Calories: 797| Carbs: 6 grams | Fats: 70 grams

INGREDIENTS:

- 4 oz./110g celery stalks
- 2 scallions
- ½ lemon, zest, and juice
- ½ cup/125ml mayonnaise
- 1 teaspoon Dijon mustard
- 4eggs
- 5 oz./150g tuna in olive oil
- 6 oz./175g Romaine lettuce
- 4 oz./110g cherry tomatoes
- 2 tablespoon olive oil
- salt and pepper to taste

INSTRUCTIONS:

1. Chop celery and onions. In a medium bowl, add lemon, mayonnaise and mustard, together with a tuna. Stir and season with salt and pepper. Set aside.

2. Add eggs to a pan and add the water to cover the eggs. Bring to a boil and let steam for 5-6 minutes if you want it to be mild or medium or 8-10 minutes

3. if you want it to be firm.

4. When done, immediately put in ice-cold water to make the egg to peel more easily. Divide them into wedges or halves.

5. Layer the tuna and egg mixture on the romaine lettuce bed. Add the tomatoes and olive oil at the top.

6. Season with salt and pepper.

KETO TEX-MEX BURGER PLATE

Servings: 2| Total Time: 15 minutes

Nutrition Information

Calories: 850| Carbs: 6 grams | Fats: 74 grams

INGREDIENTS:

- 2/3 lb/300g   beef
- 1 tablespoon Tex-Mex or taco seasoning
- 4 tablespoon olive oil
- salt and pepper
- 1oz./30g sliced Pepper Jack cheese or Mexican cheese or any other cheese
- 1 avocado
- 2 oz./50g lettuce
- 2 tablespoon pickled jalapeños
- 1/3 cup/75ml sour cream

INSTRUCTIONS:

1. Mix beef and seasoning. Make a burger per each meal(serving).

2. Roast the burgers in half of the olive oil on each side at medium heat for 3-4 minutes until the burger is light pink or fried all over, which you prefer. Salt and pepper to taste.

3. Place the hamburger with cheese, avocado, lettuce, jalapeños, and sour cream. Sprinkle with leftover olive oil.

KETO TURKEY WITH CREAM-CHEESE SAUCE

Servings: 4| Total Time: 25 minutes

Nutrition Information

Calories: 815| Carbs: 7 grams | Fats: 67 grams

INGREDIENTS:

- 2 tablespoon butter
- 1½ lbs/650g turkey breast
- Salt and pepper to taste
- 7 oz./200g cream cheese
- 1 tablespoon sauce of tamari soy
- 1½ oz./40g capers
- 2 cups/475g crème fraîche or heavy whipping cream

INSTRUCTIONS:

1. Preheat oven to 350 degrees Fahrenheit(175 degrecs Celsius).

2. Melt half of the butter in a large frying pan, over medium heat. Squeeze the turkey gently, then cook until golden brown. When the turkey is cooked through and has an internal temperature of at least 165 degrees F (74 degrees C), put it on a plate and tent using a foil

3. Pour turkey slices into a small pot. Stir with cream and cheese. Stir and raise to a light boil. Reduce heat and let thicken.

4. Add soy sauce, then season to taste with salt and pepper.

5. Heat the remaining butter over high heat, in a medium pan. Quickly sauté the capers until crispy.

6. Serve the turkey with capers and sauce.

BAKED MINI BELL PEPPERS

Servings: 4| Total Time: 35 minutes

Nutrition Information

Calories: 412| Carbs: 6 grams | Fats: 37 grams

INGREDIENTS:

- 8 oz./225g mini bell peppers
- 1 oz./30g air-dried chorizo, chopped
- 1 tablespoon fresh thyme or fresh cilantro, chopped
- 8 oz./225g cream cheese
- ½ tablespoon mild chipotle paste
- 2 tablespoon olive oil
- 4 oz./110g(225ml) shredded cheese

INSTRUCTIONS:

1. Set the oven at 200 degrees Celsius (325 degrees Fahrenheit) Lengthwise split the bell peppers and remove the core and then add chopped horizo herbs

2. In a small bowl, add the cream cheese, spices and oil. Add the chorizo and herbs. Stir until smooth.

3. fill inside the pepper with mixture and place in a dish

4. Sprinkle the top with shredded cheese. Bake 15-20 minutes in the oven, or until the cheese melts and turns golden brown.

KETO LAMB CHOPS WITH HERB BUTTER

Servings: 4| Total Time: 15 minutes

Nutrition Information

Calories: 723| Carbs: 0.3 grams | Fats: 62 grams

INGREDIENTS:

- ◆ 8 chops of lamb
- ◆ 1 tablespoon butter
- ◆ salt and pepper to taste
- ◆ 1 tablespoon olive oil

For serving

- ◆ 4 oz./110g herb butter
- ◆ 1 lemon, in wedges

INSTRUCTIONS:

1. Allow the chops to reach the room temperature before they are grilled. Meat should not be cold when its cooked, or it does not have a nice brown surface.

2. Season with salt and pepper.

3. If you are using a frying pan, fry in butter and some olive oil. If you are grilling, brush on some olive oil before placing it on the grill.

4. Fry for 3-4 minutes, depending on the thickness of the chops. thicker chops need more baking time. However, it is good for a lamb to have a little pink inside.

5. Serve with butter and lemon wedges.

KETO CHICKEN AND CABBAGE PLATE

Servings: 2| Total Time: 5 minutes

Nutrition Information

Calories: 1041| Carbs: 7 grams | Fats: 91 grams

INGREDIENTS:

- 7 oz./200g fresh green cabbage
- 1 lb/450g rotisserie chicken
- 1 tablespoon olive oil
- ½ cup/125ml mayonnaise
- ½ red onion
- salt and pepper to taste

INSTRUCTIONS:

1. Use a sharp knife to cut the cabbage, and place it on a plate.

2. Chop the onion and add it with a rotisserie chicken and a lot of mayonnaise.

3. Drizzle the oil over the cabbages and season with salt and pepper.

SPICY KETO DEVILED EGGS

Servings: 6| Total Time: 20 minutes

Nutrition Information

Calories: 200| Carbs: 1 grams | Fats: 19 grams

INGREDIENTS:

- ♦ 6 eggs
- ♦ ½ cup/125ml mayonnaise
- ♦ ¼ teaspoon salt
- ♦ 1 tablespoon red curry paste
- ♦ ½ tablespoon/5g poppy seeds

INSTRUCTIONS:

1. Put the eggs in a saucepan with cold water (water will cover the eggs). Bring without a lid to a boil. Have the eggs boil for about 8 minutes, then simmer. Quickly cool them off in ice-cold water.

2. Remove the shells from the egg. split the eggs in half and cut both ends. Separate the yolk of the egg, and put it in a pot.

3. Place egg whites on a large plate and let them stay in the refrigerator.

4. Mix together the curry, mayonnaise and egg yolks until smooth. Season with salt. Take egg whites out of the fridge and apply the batter.

5. Sprinkle the seeds and serve.

KETO HALLOUMI CHEESE AND AVOCADO PLATE

Servings: 2| Total Time: 15 minutes

Nutrition Information

Calories: 1112| Carbs: 12 grams | Fats: 100 grams

INGREDIENTS:

- ◆ 10 oz./275g halloumi cheese
- ◆ 2 tablespoon butter
- ◆ 2 tablespoon pistachio nuts
- ◆ salt and pepper to taste
- ◆ 2 avocados
- ◆ ¼ cucumber
- ◆ 1/3 cup/75ml sour cream
- ◆ 2tablespoon olive oil
- ◆ ¼ lemon (optional)

INSTRUCTIONS:

1. Cut the cheese into pieces then cook over medium heat in butter until golden. Turn them to each side for a few minutes.

2. Serve with avocado, cucumber, sour cream, pistachios, and lemon.

3. Sprinkle the oil over the vegetables. To taste, season with salt and pepper.

KETO PROSCIUTTO-WRAPPED ASPARAGUS WITH GOAT CHEESE

Servings: 4| Total Time: 25 minutes

Nutrition Information

Calories: 222| Carbs: 1 grams | Fats: 19 grams

INGREDIENTS:

- ◆ 12 pieces of green asparagus
- ◆ 2 oz./50g prosciutto, slices
- ◆ 5 oz./150g goat cheese
- ◆ ¼ teaspoon ground black pepper
- ◆ 2 tablespoon olive oil

INSTRUCTIONS:

1. Preheat oven to 225 degrees C (450 degrees Fahrenheit), ideally with broiler feature.

2. Trim and wash the asparagus.

3. Cut the cheese into 12 slices and then divide each slice into two.

4. Cut the slices of prosciutto into two pieces and wrap each slice around asparagus and two pieces of cheese. Then place all together in a baking pan covered with parchment paper. Add pepper and olive oil.

5. Place the baking saucepan in the oven until golden brown for about 15 minutes.

KETO OVEN-BAKED BRIE CHEESE

Servings: 4| Total Time: 15 minutes

Nutrition Information

Calories: 342| Carbs: 1 grams | Fats: 31 grams

INGREDIENTS:

- 2 oz./50g pecans or walnuts, chopped
- 1 garlic clove, minced
- 1 tablespoon fresh rosemary, chopped
- 1tablespoon olive oil
- 9 oz./255g Brie cheese or Camembert cheese
- salt and pepper to taste

INSTRUCTIONS:

1. Preheat oven to 200 degrees Celsius (400 degrees Fahrenheit).

2. Place the cheeses on a sheet pan covered with parchment paper or in the small cooking pan as you prefer.

3. Combine and mix the herbs nuts and garlic with olive oil in a small bowl. Garnish with salt and pepper.

4. Put the nut mixture on the cheese and leave them for about 10-12 minutes until you get soft and warm cheese and nuts are toasted enough. Then serve it!

SNACKS AND DESSERTS

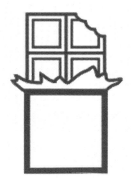

SPICY KETO ROASTED NUTS

Servings: 6| Total Time: 15 minutes

Nutrition Information

Calories: 285| Carbs: 2 grams | Fats: 30 grams

INGREDIENTS:

- 1 teaspoon ground cumin
- 1 teaspoon salt
- 8 oz./225g pecans or almonds or walnuts
- 1 teaspoon paprika powder or chilli powder
- 1 tablespoon olive oil or coconut oil

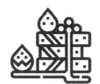

INSTRUCTIONS:

1. Combine all the ingredients in a medium saucepan and steam over medium heat to warm up the almonds.

2. Let it be cooled down and serve with a drink. Store in a container and cover with a lid at room temperature.

KETO RANCH DIP

Servings: 8| Total Time: 15 minutes

Nutrition Information

Calories: 241| Carbs: 1 grams | Fats: 26 grams

INGREDIENTS:

- ♦ 1 cup/225ml mayonnaise
- ♦ ½ cup/125ml crème fraîche or sour cream
- ♦ 2 tablespoon ranch seasoning

INSTRUCTIONS:

1. Combine the ingredients in a bowl, then place for at least 15 minutes in the fridge.Serve as a separate dish or as a salad dressing.

KETO BLUE-CHEESE DRESSING

Servings: 4| Total Time: 10 minutes

Nutrition Information

Calories: 460| Carbs: 4 grams | Fats: 44 grams

INGREDIENTS:

- ½ cup/125ml heavy whipping cream
- salt and pepper to taste
- ¾ cup/175ml Greek yoghurt
- 2 tablespoon parsley, chopped
- 5 oz./150g blue cheese
- ½ cup/125ml mayonnaise

INSTRUCTIONS:

1. Put the cheese in a medium bowl, and cut it into large pieces using a fork. Add yoghurt, mayonnaise and heavy whipped cream, mix to combine.

2. Let them sit for a couple of minutes. Add pepper, salt and parsley.

CAPRESE SNACK

Servings: 4| Total Time: 5 minutes

Nutrition Information

Calories: 218| Carbs: 3 grams | Fats: 14 grams

INGREDIENTS:

- 8 oz./225g mozzarella, mini cheese balls
- 2 tablespoon green pesto
- salt and pepper to taste
- 8 oz./225g cherry tomatoes

INSTRUCTIONS:

1. Cut tomatoes and mozzarella balls in half. Stir while adding pesto

2. Salt and pepper to taste.

CINNAMON AND CARDAMOM FAT BOMBS

Servings: 10| Total Time: 45 minutes

Nutrition Information

Calories: 90| Carbs: 0.4 grams | Fats: 10 grams

INGREDIENTS:

- ◆ 3 oz./75g unsalted butter
- ◆ ½ cup/50g(125ml) coconut, shredded
- ◆ ¼ teaspoon ground cardamom (green)
- ◆ ½ teaspoon vanilla extract
- ◆ ¼ tsp cinnamon

INSTRUCTIONS:

1. Let the melt to room temperature.

2. Carefully roast the chopped coconut over medium-high heat until light brown. Let it cool.

3. In a small bowl, add half the shredded coconut, butter, spices. Freeze the mixture in the refrigerator for 5-10 minutes, until relatively solid.

4. Shape into walnut-sized balls. Then spin the balls into the remaining shredded coconut and store it in the freezer or refrigerator.

COFFEE WITH CREAM

Servings: 1| Total Time: 5 minutes

Nutrition Information

Calories: 202| Carbs: 2 grams | Fats: 21 grams

INGREDIENTS:

- ¾ cup/175ml coffee, brewed
- ¼ cup/60ml heavy whipping cream

INSTRUCTIONS:

1. Make your own coffee the way you like. Pour the cream into a small saucepan and heat until frothy.

2. Pour warm cream into a large cup, add coffee and stir. Serve immediately with nuts or dark chocolate.

KETO HOT CHOCOLATE

Servings: 1| Total Time: 5 minutes

Nutrition Information

Calories: 216| Carbs: 1 grams | Fats: 23 grams

INGREDIENTS:

- ◆ 1 oz./30g unsalted butter
- ◆ 1/4 teaspoon vanilla extract
- ◆ 1 tablespoon/5g cocoa powder
- ◆ 2½ teaspoon/10g powdered erythritol
- ◆ 1cup/225ml boiling water

INSTRUCTIONS:

1. Place the ingredients on a tall beaker in order to use immersion mixer and mix only for 15-20 seconds until you can see foam on top of the beaker.

2. Mix for 15-20 seconds or until there is a good foam on top.

LOW-CARB CHIA PUDDING

Servings: 1| Total Time: 5 minutes

Nutrition Information

Calories: 568| Carbs: 8 grams | Fats: 56 grams

INGREDIENTS:

- ◆ 1 cup/225ml unsweetened, canned coconut milk or unsweetened almond milk
- ◆ 2 tablespoon/25g chia seeds
- ◆ ½ teaspoon vanilla extract

INSTRUCTIONS:

1. Mix all of the ingredients together in a container until smooth.

2. Set in the refrigerator for at least 4 hours. Make sure the pudding has thickened, and the chia seeds are gelled.

3. Serve the pudding with cream, coconut milk or some fresh or frozen berries.

BONUS (VEGETARIAN RECIPES)

BONUS (VEGETARIAN RECIPES)

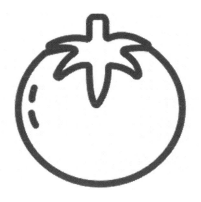

COLESLAW

Servings: 4| Total Time: 15 minutes

Nutrition Information

Calories: 209| Carbs: 3 grams | Fats: 21 grams

INGREDIENTS:

- ◆ 1 tablespoon Dijon mustard
- ◆ 1 teaspoon salt
- ◆ ½ lb/225g green cabbage
- ◆ ½ cup/125ml vegan mayonnaise
- ◆ 1 pinch fennel seeds (optional)
- ◆ 1 pinch of pepper
- ◆ ½lemon, juice

INSTRUCTIONS:

1. Use a food processor or sharp cheese slicer to remove the core and smash the cabbage.

2. place the cabbage in a medium-sized bowl. Add salt and lemon juice and leave it on the oven to boil for 10 minutes and let the cabbage melt a little. You shouldn't add any additional liquid

3. Mix optional cabbage, mayonnaise, and mustard.

4. Season of Taste.

LOW-CARB CAULIFLOWER RICE

Servings: 4| Total Time: 20 minutes

Nutrition Information

Calories: 193| Carbs: 5 grams | Fats: 18 grams

INGREDIENTS:

- ◆ 1½ lbs/650g cauliflower
- ◆ ½ teaspoon salt
- ◆ ½ teaspoon turmeric (optional)
- ◆ 3 oz./75g butter or coconut oil

INSTRUCTIONS:

1. Use a grater to shred the entire cauliflower head

2. add coconut oil or melt butter in a frying pan. Add the cauliflower and cook for 5 to 10 minutes over medium heat or until slightly softened

3. While frying adds salt and turmeric(optional).

RUTABAGA CURLS

Servings: 4| Total Time: 30 minutes

Nutrition Information

Calories: 227| Carbs: 11 grams | Fats: 18 grams

INGREDIENTS:

- 1 tablespoon salt
- 1/3 cup/75ml olive oil
- 1 tablespoon paprika powder or chilli powder
- 1½ lbs/650g rutabaga

INSTRUCTIONS:

1. Heat the oven to 225 degrees Celsius (450 degrees Fahrenheit).Peel the rutabaga and cut into pieces that you can use with your spiralizer. You can also use a sharp knife if you don't have a spiralizer.

2. Put in a plastic bowl or bag then pour over other ingredients and stir or shake thoroughly.

3. Layer over a baking sheet, then cook 10 minutes in the oven.

4. You can serve it with the main course of your choice!

KETO KOHLSLAW

Servings: 4| Total Time: 15 minutes

Nutrition Information

Calories: 405| Carbs: 3 grams | Fats: 41 grams

INGREDIENTS:

- ◆ fresh parsley (optional)
- ◆ salt and pepper to taste
- ◆ 1 lb/450g kohlrabi
- ◆ 1 cup/225ml vegan mayonnaise

INSTRUCTIONS:

1. Peel Kohlrabi. Be sure to remove the hard and wooden parts. Shred-it finely chop place it into a bowl.

2. Add fresh herbs and mayonnaise.

3. Salt and pepper to taste.

SPICY ALMOND AND SEED MIX

Servings: 10| Total Time: 15 minutes

Nutrition Information

Calories: 234| Carbs: 3 grams | Fats: 21 grams

INGREDIENTS:

- 2tablespoon coconut oil or olive oil
- 1 tablespoon ground cumin or crushed fennel seeds
- 5 oz./150g almonds
- 4 oz./110g(200ml) pumpkin seeds
- 4 oz./110g(175ml) sunflower seeds
- 1tablespoon chilli paste
- ½ teaspoon salt

INSTRUCTIONS:

1. In a large frying pan, heat oil and add chilli first.

2. Add almonds and seeds you should stir it hard

3. Sauté for a few minutes of salt and sauce, but beware because the almonds and seeds are very sensitive to heat and they should not be burned.

4. Let it cool and put in a glass jar.Serve as a snack.

OVEN-BAKED RUTABAGA WEDGES

Servings: 4| Total Time: 25 minutes

Nutrition Information

Calories: 167| Carbs: 7 grams | Fats: 14 grams

INGREDIENTS:

- ◆ salt and pepper to taste
- ◆ ¼cup/60ml olive oil
- ◆ 1 teaspoon chilli powder or paprika powder
- ◆ 1 lb/450g rutabaga

INSTRUCTIONS:

1. Heat the oven to 400 degrees Fahrenheit (200 degrees Celsius).

2. Wash the rosettes and peel it. Smaller roots are cooked faster in the oven.

3. Split into wedges, and spread over a baking sheet.salt and pepper. Sprinkle over olive oil and mix properly.

4. Place in the oven and bake for 20 minutes or until well-coloured. Use a knife to check if they are ready. They bake faster than the bottom, so pay attention.

5. Serve with the meat or fish you want.

ROASTED POINTED CABBAGE WITH MOZZARELLA CHEESE

Servings: 4| Total Time: 40 minutes

Nutrition Information

Calories: 588| Carbs: 9 grams | Fats: 54 grams

INGREDIENTS:

- ¼teaspoon ground black pepper
- 8 oz./225g mozzarella cheese, shredded
- 2 lbs/900g cabbages
- 7 oz./200g butter
- 1 teaspoon salt
- 1 teaspoon dried rosemary

INSTRUCTIONS:

1. Heat the oven to 400 degrees Fahrenheit (200 degrees Celsius).

2. Cut the cabbage into wedges and put it in a saucepan. Add salt and pepper, and dried herbs. Paste the butter and put it in the oven for 15 minutes or until desired cabbage

3. Take it out from the oven, and add mozzarella . Again put in the oven for about 15-20 minutes until the cheese bubbles and reach good colour.

CREAMED GREEN CABBAGE

Servings: 4| Total Time: 20 minutes

Nutrition Information

Calories: 398| Carbs: 8 grams | Fats: 38 grams

INGREDIENTS:

- 1 tablespoon lemon zest
- salt and pepper to taste
- 1¼ cups/300ml heavy whipping cream
- 1½ lbs/650g grecn cabbage
- 2 oz./50g butter
- ½ cup/125ml parsley, chopped

INSTRUCTIONS:

1. Start with a food processor or sharp knife to shred the cabbage.

2. Melt the butter over medium to high heat in a frying pan. Add a few minutes of cabbage and sauté to a soft, golden brown around the edges.

3. Add heavy whipping cream and let the cabbage simmer over the lowest heat.

4. Add the parsley and lemon before serving.

5. Salt and pepper to taste.

SALAD SANDWICHES

Servings: 1| Total Time: 5 minutes

Nutrition Information

Calories: 374| Carbs: 3 grams | Fats: 34 grams

INGREDIENTS:

- ½ oz./15g butter
- 1 oz./30g Edam cheese or other cheese of your liking
- 2 oz./50g Romaine lettuce or baby gem lettuce
- ½ avocado
- 1 cherry tomatoes

INSTRUCTIONS:

1. Wash lettuce thoroughly and use it for the topping. Sprinkle butter on lettuce leaves and chop cheese, avocado, and tomatoes.

LOW-CARB CAULIFLOWER MASH

Servings: 4| Total Time: 20 minutes

Nutrition Information

Calories: 313| Carbs: 5 grams | Fats: 28 grams

INGREDIENTS:

♦ 1 lb/450g cauliflower

♦ 3 oz./75g grated Parmesan cheese

♦ 4 oz./110g butter

♦ ½ lemon, juice, and zest

♦ olive oil (optional)

INSTRUCTIONS:

1. Chop the cauliflower

2. Boil the cauliflower a few minutes in salted water, just enough for cauliflower florets are tender strain the florets in a colander and discard the water.

3. Add cauliflower with remaining ingredients to a food processor to achieve desired consistency. An immersion blender may also be used.

4. Season with salt, pepper and olive oil

DISCLAIMER

DISCLAIMER

This book contains opinions and ideas of the author and is meant to teach the reader informative and helpful knowledge while due care should be taken by the user in the application of the information provided. The instructions and strategies are possibly not right for every reader and there is no guarantee that they work for everyone. Using this book and implementing the information/recipes therein contained is explicitly your own responsibility and risk. This work with all its contents, does not guarantee correctness, completion, quality or correctness of the provided information. Misinformation or misprints cannot be completely eliminated.

Design: Natalia Design

Picture: Kiian Oksana / www.shutterstock.com

Printed in Poland
by Amazon Fulfillment
Poland Sp. z o.o., Wrocław